CHOW DOWN, SLIM UP

Beat Your Diet with Eating Right

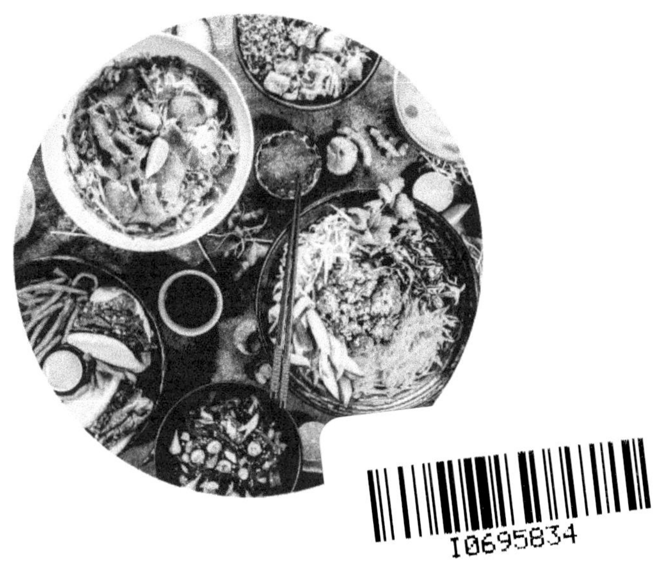

Amanda M. Brooks

Table of Content

Introduction

"Chow Down, Slim Up: Beat Your Diet with Eating Right" is a game-changing strategy for health, well-being, and long-term weight loss. This book is your guide to breaking free from the shackles of fad diets, restrictive meal plans, and the never-ending cycle of deprivation, only to gain the weight back quickly.

If you've ever been imprisoned in an endless struggle with your bathroom scale, you're not alone. The road to obtaining and maintaining a healthy weight can be difficult, filled with frustration, confusion, and countless failed attempts. It's time to break free from the diet trap and discover a liberating truth: you can eat your way to a healthier, leaner you.

In these pages, we shall present a paradigm shift that challenges current dieting thinking. Instead of condemning food or watching every calorie, we'll look at the power of making informed decisions and appreciating meals that nourish your body, mind, and spirit.

"Chow Down, Slim Up"'s fundamental premise revolves around the idea that eating healthy isn't about deprivation; it's about empowerment. It is about understanding how food affects your metabolism, hormones, and overall health. It's about enjoying delicious, nutrient-rich meals while meeting your weight-loss goals.

Throughout this trip, you will learn the secrets of a healthy metabolism, the art of mindful eating, and the science underlying long-term weight control. You'll delve into the realm of nutrient-dense foods, embrace the enchantment of balanced macronutrients, and discover how to harness the power of critical micronutrients for maximum health.

The focus of this book is not on one-size-fits-all repairs or quick fixes. Instead, it's a holistic, science-backed approach that will empower you to make decisions that are right for your individual body and lifestyle. By the end of these pages, you'll have the knowledge, resources, and inspiration to improve your relationship with food, reach your weight-loss objectives, and embark on a lifelong journey to a healthier, slimmer, and more vibrant you.

So let us go on this transformative journey together. It's time to say goodbye to diets and welcome a new way of eating well - a way that will not only help you lose those excess pounds but also empower you to succeed in every aspect of your life. "Chow Down, Slim Up" is pleased to welcome you.

Chapter 1

The Importance of Fresh, Whole Foods

Whole Foods are foods that have been processed or refined as little as possible and contain no additives such as preservatives or artificial components such as food coloring. A roasted potato, for example, is a full food, but fast mashed potatoes or packaged scalloped potatoes are not. Broiled white fish or perch, as opposed to a fish stick, would be classified as whole foods.

Whole foods have more nutrients such as fiber, minerals, and vitamins than processed meals and, when consumed in large quantities, may reduce the risk of heart disease, cancer, and type 2 diabetes. Nutrients naturally collaborate effectively within whole foods, whereas numerous processed products, such as white flour, require vitamin supplementation due to the substantial nutrient loss during processing. Nevertheless, even fortified meals fail to provide the same level of nutrition as whole foods.

Sugar is not added to whole meals. Sugar consumption is linked to an increased risk of obesity, type 2 diabetes, fatty liver disease, and heart disease. Less sugar aids in blood sugar regulation and lowers harmful fat levels. Sugar reduction is also beneficial to teeth. Sugar and refined carbohydrates in the Western diet can contribute to dental damage by feeding the plaque-causing bacteria in your mouth. The sugar and acid in ordinary soda are especially prone to deterioration.

Sugar cravings typically reduce when whole foods are consumed rather than manufactured items. Eating a well-balanced, unprocessed diet may also help reduce inflammation, which has been linked to an increased risk of heart disease and discomfort. Antioxidants are more typically found in whole foods. Antioxidants help fight free radicals, which can injure your body's cells. They can be found in all-natural foods, especially plant foods like vegetables, fruits, nuts, whole grains, and legumes.

Consuming whole meals may assist in nourishing the beneficial bacteria in your stomach. Whole fruits and vegetables, as well as whole grains, contain fiber and nourish good bacteria, which helps improve digestive health. To give even more value, try entire fermented foods like green beans.

Fiber has numerous health benefits, including improved digestive function and sensations of fullness. Fiber-rich foods include avocados, wild rice, legumes, nuts, flaxseeds, and berries. Consuming fiber through whole foods is preferable to taking a supplement since it keeps you satiated for longer and provides additional nutrients from the food itself.

Overeating has been linked to a high intake of processed and fast foods, according to a study. Sugars are not found in whole foods. Salt and flavorings are added to processed foods, which might lead to overeating.

The Power of Whole Foods in Combination

One of the most significant benefits of eating whole foods is the natural synergy of all of these nutrients. Vitamin E, selenium, and a variety of antioxidants are all present. We know that eating them in food has a variety of health benefits. However, investigations of single vitamins and minerals in supplement form have not yielded the same results. It could be a natural combination and interaction of all of these different phytochemicals and proteins that give food its health benefits. Attempting to extract and consume a single nutrient on its own may not be successful.

There's one more thing. We just do not know all of the components that make a portion of food nutritious. Nutrition research is always uncovering new dietary components that we were unaware of. Many of these do not even exist as supplements. We can't synthesize them if we don't know what they are.

Avoid Food Additives

The loss of nutrients during processing is not the only downside of eating processed foods. What is added can also be problematic. Many health-conscious consumers are concerned about the preservatives and chemicals added to processed and manufactured meals.

The most concerning additions are not preservatives, but salt, sugar, saturated and trans fats. While trans fats have received a lot of attention in recent years, salt remains vastly underappreciated. We frequently consume far too much salt, which is linked to high blood pressure and a variety of other health issues.

The calories in processed foods can quickly pile up with all of the extra fat and sugar. This results in weight gain. However, eating more healthful whole foods may help you maintain or decrease weight. Many vegetables, fruits, and grains have natural fiber, which can fill you up without adding many calories.

The Price of Whole Foods

There's another advantage to eating complete, healthful meals. Whole foods are significantly less expensive than processed foods. They are also widely available. In general, the more processed something is, the more expensive it is. A bag of healthful brown rice will be less expensive than a costly premade rice mix.

Eating healthful whole meals may have an additional cost: preparation time. It's difficult to argue that putting a processed sandwich pocket in the microwave for three minutes is less time-consuming than preparing a healthy dinner with whole-food ingredients.

You do not need to stop eating all processed meals. The idea is simply to reduce your use of processed meals while increasing your consumption of nutritious whole foods. That's not difficult, especially when it comes to snacking. Instead, eat a handful of nuts or a piece of fruit. It's no more difficult than grabbing for an energy bar; you'll even save yourself the trouble of unwrapping it.

Variety is another important aspect of a healthy diet. It's easy to get caught up in the minutiae, such as the nutritional content of specific nutritious whole meals and how much of each you require. The best recommendation is to consume a wide variety of fruits, veggies, and whole grains. It's not only simple, but it's also the greatest method to ensure you're getting all of the nutrients you require.

Eating Seasonally and Locally
Eating local, seasonal produce is good for your health, the environment, the local economy, and even your bank account.

What Counts as Seasonal Produce?
Seasonal produce includes fruits and vegetables that are accessible at different times of the year. Temperature variation throughout the year impacts the production cycles of fruits and vegetables, thus various foods grow better at different periods of the year in a given place.

According to a study published in the Proceedings of the Nutrition Society, "seasonality can be defined as either globally seasonal (i.e., produced during the natural production season but consumed anywhere in the world) or locally seasonal (i.e., produced during the natural production season and consumed within the same climatic zone)."

What Counts as Local Produce?

Global food systems have changed dramatically during the last six decades. Sixty years ago, around 70% of the produce sold in markets and grocery stores across the United States and much of Europe was cultivated, produced, and processed within 100 miles of the place of sale. Food now travels an average of 1,500 miles before it reaches a plate.

The US Food, Conservation, and Energy Act of 2008 defines local foods as agricultural food products produced locally or regionally and eaten within 400 miles of their origin or within the state in which they are produced. Nonetheless, other organizations define local foods as those produced within a 100-mile radius or a state. According to a 2015 study, most metropolitan populations in the United States could be fed by foods produced within 100 miles of them.

The Relationship Between Seasonal and Local Produce

We often eat seasonally and locally when we eat seasonally. However, many successful seasonal food retail establishments can meet demand by shipping or importing products from across the country. It is feasible to consume seasonal vegetables that were produced thousands of kilometers distant. Pumpkins, for example, are considered seasonal in the fall. However, to meet the demand for pumpkins, the United States imports around one-third of its pumpkins from Mexico. These pumpkins are considered seasonal in the United States, but the distance they must travel to get there negates some of the economic and environmental benefits of eating vegetables grown in your region.

In other words, because of importation, you can eat seasonal foods while not eating locally. With the use of technologies such as greenhouses, it is also possible to eat non-seasonal local foods. However, neither of these strategies takes advantage of the ecological and economic benefits of consuming locally grown, seasonal foods.

What is Seasonal Eating?

When you 'Eat the Seasons,' you eat food at the times of year that nature meant for us. Each season has its prime produce, which is when it is at its peak in terms of size, taste, nutritional content, and overall goodness. For example, root vegetables such as carrots, parsnips, and potatoes provide warmth during the gloomy winter months but are considered too heavy for the brighter summer months. Fresh greens and tomatoes, on the other hand, are more likely to meet your body's requirement to be active in the sun.

Seasonal eating has two key advantages. To begin with, unseasonally cultivated crops have a higher carbon footprint due to the extra heating, lighting, water, and, in the worst-case scenario, pesticides required to grow them out of season. Second, it is claimed that consuming seasonal produce is more likely to be fresher, consumed closer to harvesting, and higher in nutritional content, as several antioxidants such as Vitamin C, folate, and carotenes degrade rapidly when stored for extended periods.

Reasons to Eat Seasonal, Local Food
Including more locally grown and seasonal foods in your diet offers numerous advantages for you, your community, and the environment. Here are some of the reasons we believe you should eat seasonally and locally.

1. Local Produce Is Healthy: A fresh bowl of fruits and vegetables is vital for healthy health. We labor all day to have a healthy and fit life, and we may do so by simply chewing on the nutritious fruits and veggies that complement our health so beautifully. The best aspect is that they are so readily available that we may purchase the best fruits and vegetables from local merchants.

2. Diet diversity. Eating seasonal foods not only guarantees that we are getting the most nutritious meals, but it also adds diversity to our diet. Instead of eating apples all year, try strawberries in the late spring, peaches and apricots in the summer, watermelons and melons in the early fall, and persimmons and pomegranates in the winter.

3. It benefits your community: When you buy locally grown food, your money stays

within to help the farmers and communities.

4. It's simpler to understand what you're getting: When it comes to food, our globalized food system provides us with a wealth of options and ease. However, extending the distance between where food is grown and processed makes obtaining information about how it was created more difficult. Knowing where your food comes from is the simplest way to get to know it.

5. You can assist. Stop Wasting Food! : The longer food is stored and transported, the more likely it will spoil and go to waste. More than half of all food waste happens somewhere in the supply chain. Buying locally and seasonally can help reduce the likelihood of food waste before it reaches the shops.

6. There will be no post-harvest treatment. Chemicals may be used to keep food fresh

during shipping. Locally cultivated fruits and vegetables do not require treatment. Your farmer can also teach you about harvesting methods and food handling practices. Do they use chlorinated water to rinse the greens? Do they use a treatment to keep potatoes, onions, and garlic from sprouting? Is the apple waxed?

The Importance of Seasonal and Local Food.

1. Spring: Spring fruits and vegetables are high in vitamins and minerals, which are necessary for a healthy diet. Spring provides a pleasant wind at night and sunshine during the day. Typically, you can quickly develop a cold or flu if you do not consume anti-allergenic foods.

    - Cherries, jackfruit, avocado, pineapple, cantaloupe, and apricots are among the fruits.

- Beetroot, garlic, spring onion, carrot, cabbage, and beans are among the vegetables.

2. Autumn: Autumn, often known as fall, is neither cool nor hot. With the onset of fall, the leaves begin to change color. This is not a good season for farming because there has been no rain and it is a sort of dry season. Autumn fruits and vegetables, on the other hand, are still high in vitamins and minerals.

   - Sweet lime, custard apple, black Jamun, guava, bananas, and pears are among the fruits.

   - Mushrooms, lettuce, potatoes, sweet corn, and sweet potatoes are among the vegetables.

3. Summer fruits and vegetables help you stay full and are important for digestion. They have fiber, micronutrients, and water in them. In the summer, we tend to spend more time outside and sweat more, so it's critical to

drink plenty of water and consume water-rich foods like watermelons to stay hydrated.

- Watermelons, strawberries, mangoes, plums, lychees, and rambutans are among the fruits.
- Cluster beans, zucchini, cucumber, bottle gourd, brinjal, and tomatoes are among the vegetables.

4. Winter: The severity of winter varies depending on where you live or travel between December and February. While the south of India offers mild weather with manageable temperatures, the north may be bitterly cold. And with winter comes a new set of illnesses and infections to protect ourselves from, so eating fresh and local foods is even more important. Winter vegetables and fruits are high in nutrients, minerals, and flavor.

- Apples, oranges, lemons, kiwi, papaya, dates, and grapes are examples of fruits.

- Ash gourd, bitter gourd, spinach, turnip, cauliflower, and pumpkins are among the vegetables.

Shopping Techniques for Nutrient-Rich Foods

As a dietitian, I am well aware that for many people, grocery shopping may be a frightening and overwhelming process. Many of my patients, for example, don't know where to start in the grocery store and are unsure of which foods to add to their cart. Furthermore, with apparently unlimited food options accessible — frequently in deceptive packaging — it can be difficult to tell which foods are genuinely healthy and which should be avoided.

The grocery shop is the first step in a healthy diet. In every aisle, choose nutrient-rich foods. For relatively fewer calories, nutrient-rich food provides more vitamins, minerals, and other nutrients. In almost every aisle of the supermarket, you may find foods that are high in nutrients.

Pick out a range of fruits and vegetables in different colors from the produce section. Also in the frozen section, there are lots of nutritious choices. Juice and canned foods should be avoided as they tend to contain greater levels of sugar and sodium and less fiber. Choose fruits and vegetables that are at least three to five distinct colors apart. Greater nutritional diversity will result from this. Look for lower-fat foods in the chilled section, such as yogurt with reduced or no fat, soy milk, skim or 1% milk, and other dairy alternatives.

Because deli meat contains nitrates and sodium, it is better to buy fresh, lean meats and poultry at the butcher counter. If you're buying frozen meat, make sure there is just one component in the meal you're buying by reading the nutrition information or ingredients. In frozen foods, there are frequently unmarked sources of sodium, which can increase the weight and raise the price. Look for fish like salmon and trout, as well as shellfish like shrimp and crab, that are high in omega-3 fatty acids at the seafood counter.

Wild Pacific salmon and trout are your best options if you want to eat fish with minimal mercury levels. Shrimp is a greater source of cholesterol and typically contains high levels of sodium, so it's crucial to be aware of this if you eat it frequently. For confirmation, once more, consult the D.V. percentage listed on the nutrition information.

Brown rice, bulgur, quinoa, and barley are examples of whole, unprocessed grains that you should choose while shopping for grains. Look for what I refer to as "Single Ingredient Foods" most frequently. Choose whole grains and variants with more fiber when you buy bread and cereal. Make sure your product is made entirely of whole grains, not merely "made with whole grains" or "multigrain," as manufacturers are getting craftier. These are posh marketing terms that occasionally deceive. The sugar and sodium content of grain products should also be considered because these two nutrients are sometimes excessively high.

Look for legumes like black beans and chickpeas in the inner aisles, as well as lentils. Due to the lack of additional sodium, dried beans, and lentils are preferred. Because they appear to have less oligosaccharide after being cooked, they are also more readily accepted in terms of digestion by many people.

Last but not least, seek out raw or dry-roasted nuts and seeds including walnuts, almonds, pumpkin, and sunflower seeds. These fats are good for you and are packed with trace elements and minerals. When it comes to calories, it is simple to consume too many of these healthy foods, therefore it's crucial to know how many there are before you eat any.

Make a grocery list of healthful foods
While some people can go grocery shopping without a list or a notion of the meals they'll prepare over the next week, the majority of people need some kind of plan. If you are easily distracted at stores or are unsure of where to start, it is a good idea to have a shopping list or a weekly meal with you.

For many consumers, a shopping list is a crucial tool. You can be reminded of the things you need and keep on task with its assistance. Furthermore, research suggests that grocery lists may aid in your decision-making while shopping for healthier options. Nevertheless, what is on a "healthy" grocery list?

When making your shopping list, it can be useful to divide it into categories like nonstarchy and starchy vegetables, fruits, beans and grains, nuts and seeds, proteins, frozen foods, dairy and nondairy replacements, drinks, condiments, and other miscellaneous products.

A healthy grocery cart might include the following items:
- cauliflower, broccoli, leeks, sweet peppers, onions, bell peppers, greens, and asparagus are examples of non-starchy vegetables.
- Fruits include avocados, oranges, bananas, apples, grapefruit, lemons, blueberries, and bananas.
- Eggs, fish, poultry, ground turkey, and tofu are all sources of protein.
- Potatoes, winter squash, and other starchy veggies

- Grain and legume selections include quinoa, oats, brown rice, dry black beans, buckwheat, red lentils, barley, and farro.
- Pumpkin seeds, macadamia nuts, almonds, and natural peanut butter are some of the nuts and nut butter that are available.
- Salmon, sardines, beans, pumpkin puree, chopped tomatoes, and marinara sauce are a few examples of things that can be purchased.
- Salad dressing, avocado oil, salsa, apple cider vinegar, balsamic vinegar, dried spices, honey, and maple syrup are just a few of the oils and condiments available.
- Products that are both dairy and vegan include full-fat Greek yogurt, cheddar cheese, goat cheese, cashew milk, and coconut yogurt.
- Trail mix, hummus, unsweetened dried fruit, and dark chocolate chips are some examples of healthy snacks.

- frozen kale, frozen prawns, and frozen raspberries are some examples of frozen foods.
- Caffeine, herbal tea bags, and unsweetened seltzer water are some examples of beverages.

Even though this list isn't definitive or thorough, it might serve as a broad roadmap for shopping excursions. Naturally, a nutritious, well-balanced diet also has room for your favorite foods. It's not necessary to fully forgo items like cookies, ice cream, and chips that are seen as less healthful.

Sadly, the majority of supermarkets are not built to promote a healthy diet. Instead, they are arranged to persuade you to buy particular, occasionally unhealthy things. For instance, supermarkets frequently run promotions and set up displays for ultra-processed goods like upscale snacks and soft beverages. A plan will make it less likely for you to become sidetracked by advertisements and sales. Just remember to only buy the things on your list. Try to just shop for groceries when you are not hungry to prevent making impulsive purchases.

Chapter 2

Understanding Your Metabolism

Metabolism is the sum of all events that occur within each cell of the body and supply energy to the organism. Energy from food and beverages is transformed into energy, which powers all of the critical processes that take place inside the body continually and allows for life and regular functioning. Factors such as gender, height, age, activity, food, and disease all have an impact on the body's rate of energy production, which is measured in calories.

Some people attribute their weight gain to how their bodies convert food into energy, often known as metabolism. They think their metabolism is moving too slowly. But is that the true cause? Is it possible to speed up the procedure if this is the case?

True, the rate at which the body digests food is related to weight. However, weight gain is rarely brought on by a slow metabolism. The amount of energy the body needs to function does depend on metabolism. But a person's diet, amount of alcohol consumption, and level of exercise all affect their weight.

Food is turned into energy through the metabolic process.

The process through which the body transforms food and liquids into energy is referred to as metabolism. In this process, oxygen and calories from food and liquids mix to create the energy that the body needs. Even while the body is at rest, energy is still needed for proper operation. This includes breathing, sending blood through the body's circulatory system, preserving the proper balance of hormones, and creating and repairing new cells. The basal metabolic rate, also known as basal metabolism, is the quantity of calories that a body burns while at rest.

The fundamental factor of basal metabolic rate is muscle mass. Additionally affecting basal metabolic rate are body size and composition. Larger or more muscular persons burn more calories even while at rest.

Metabolic rate and weight loss

You might want to attribute a medical condition to your sluggish metabolism and weight gain. However, a medical condition seldom slows metabolism enough to result in appreciable weight gain. Weight gain can result from Cushing syndrome and hypothyroidism, a disorder marked by an underactive thyroid gland. These unique circumstances exist.

Weight gain is influenced by numerous variables. Most likely, they include genetics, hormones, diet, and lifestyle elements including stress, sleep, and physical activity. When you consume more calories than you burn or consume less calories than you burn, you gain weight.

Some people seem to lose weight more quickly and easily than others. To lose weight, one must, however, burn more calories than they take in. The fact remains that calories are important. Either consume fewer calories or exercise more if you want to lose weight. Also possible are both.

The study of metabolism and physical activity
Although your basal metabolic rate is something you cannot easily change, you can control how many calories you burn through exercise. You burn more calories when you walk around more. People who seem to have a quick metabolism may be more active and fidgety than they appear to be.

The following activities are recommended by the Physical Activity Guidelines for Americans to burn more calories:

- Aerobic activity: As a general rule, strive to engage in at least 30 minutes of moderate physical activity each day. If you want to lose weight, keep it off, or reach particular fitness objectives, you might need to exercise more.

- Moderate aerobic exercise includes activities like swimming, mowing the grass, riding a bike, and walking quickly. Exercises that are vigorously aerobic include running, strenuous yard labor, and aerobic dancing.

- Exercising your muscles: Exercises for strength training should be done for all main muscle groups at least twice per week. Strength training can be done using weight machines, your body weight, heavy bags, resistance tubing or paddles in the water, or sports like rock climbing.

What Role Does Metabolism Play Here?

Catabolism and anabolism are the two fundamental chemical processes involved in metabolism. While catabolic reactions control the breakdown of food to provide energy, anabolic reactions use that energy to construct larger molecules. Life requires both catabolic and anabolic reactions to function.

For the purpose of supplying energy, molecules are broken down during catabolism. This includes breaking down macronutrients (proteins, carbs, and fats) into simpler forms to provide energy and the basic building blocks for growth.

Anabolism is the synthesis of all substances that the cells require. This includes development and repair, which require energy from our diet. The majority of the energy (calories) we consume daily is used to maintain catabolic and anabolic reactions going in the body, while a lesser portion is used to power activities.

Components Of Metabolism

There are four main components of metabolism:

- Basal Metabolic Rate (BMR)
- Thermic Effect of Food (TEF)
- Exercise Activity Thermogenesis (EAT)
- Non-Exercise Activity Thermogenesis (NEAT)

BMR + TEF + EAT + NEAT = TDEE

Each component of metabolism consumes energy and contributes to our total daily energy expenditure (TDEE), also referred to as your metabolism.

Basal Metabolic Rate

The amount of energy consumed by the body at rest or for the most fundamental life-sustaining tasks is known as your basal metabolic rate (BMR). Even when you are sleeping, your body requires energy for breathing, circulation, nutrient digestion, hormone regulation, and cell formation. The body's BMR accounts for the majority of the energy expended daily, accounting for around 70% of total daily energy expenditure. BMR is affected by several parameters, including gender, age, height, fat mass, fat-free mass, and hormones.

The terms basal metabolic rate (BMR) and resting metabolic rate (RMR) are sometimes used interchangeably, however, there is a subtle distinction between the two. Both BMR and RMR quantify the amount of energy - in calories - the body requires to stay alive and function properly; however, RMR takes into account additional low-effort daily activities in addition to essential bodily processes. Eating and visiting the restroom are examples of low-effort tasks. As a result, there is around a 10% discrepancy between your BMR and RMR, because RMR accounts for slightly more energy expended each day.

Thermal Effect of Food

The energy expended to digest, metabolize, absorb, and store food is referred to as the thermic effect of food (TEF), also known as diet-induced thermogenesis. TEF accounts for about 10% of your daily energy expenditure; however, it is impacted by age, meal timing, and the macronutrient composition of your meal. Each macronutrient - protein, carbohydrate, and fat – necessitates a specific amount of energy (TEF) to be digested by the body, which can be stated as a percentage of the energy that they contain:

- Fat thermic impact = 0-3%
- Carbohydrate thermogenic action = 5-10%
- Protein has a thermogenic impact of 20-30%.

Protein has the largest thermic effect of the three macronutrients, which means that the body uses more energy to break down 1 gram of protein than 1 gram of carbohydrate or fat.

Exercise Activity Thermogenesis

The energy expended by the body during physical action is referred to as exercise activity thermogenesis (EAT). EAT accounts for periods of deliberate exercise, such as going for a run, lifting weights, swimming, or working out. Because it is affected by how active you are each day, EAT changes most of all metabolic components and can contribute for anywhere from 5% to 30% of your total daily expenditure depending on the individual.

Non-Exercise Activity Thermogenesis

Non-exercise activity thermogenesis (NEAT) refers to the energy expended for activities other than sleeping, eating, and sports-like exercise. This includes energy wasted while walking to the restroom, standing, cooking, cleaning, and fidgeting. Your NEAT is responsible for about 15% of your entire daily energy expenditure.

How Does Weight Impact Metabolism?

Metabolism has a direct influence on weight reduction and gain. When we consume more energy than we require for metabolism and physical exercise, the surplus is generally stored as adipose tissue, often known as body fat. When less energy is consumed than is required for metabolism and physical activity, the body will use previously stored energy. This relationship between "energy in" and "energy out" is referred to as energy balance, which is governed by thermodynamic rules and determines whether weight is lost, gained, or remains constant.

Does Diet Have An Effect On Metabolism?

Because the thermic effect of food (TEF) is part of your total daily energy expenditure (TDEE), your diet affects your metabolism. Your meal's macronutrient composition has a direct impact on how much energy your body expends to digest it. Protein has the highest thermic effect of any food, 10% to 30% higher than carbohydrates or fat; thus, protein-rich foods can help to increase your metabolism; While evidence is limited, some research suggests that high-carb meals produce a greater thermic effect than high-fat meals.

Does Muscle Help With Metabolism?

Because body composition or an individual's muscle-to-fat ratio influences basal metabolic rate (BMR), increasing muscle mass increases metabolism. entire lean mass, or your body's entire weight minus fat mass, requires a lot of energy to maintain. Individuals with more lean muscle mass will generally have a faster metabolic rate than those with less lean muscle mass.

Exercise Improves Metabolism?

Because exercise activity thermogenesis (EAT) influences total daily energy expenditure (TDEE), or the total number of calories burned each day, it has a direct impact on metabolism. While BMR accounts for the majority of the energy expended by the body, exercise is still vital to metabolism and overall health. Exercise not only immediately increases energy expenditure during the activity, but the increase in metabolic activity caused by exercise can outlast your session. Your metabolism may continue to burn calories at rest as a result of increased oxygen consumption after workouts, a process known as excess post-exercise oxygen consumption, or EPOC, depending on the length and intensity of your physical activity. Interestingly, while aerobic activities such as jogging, cycling, or swimming burn more calories during exercise, anaerobic activities like as weight lifting or interval training, which have a greater EPOC, can help you waste more energy after exercising. Your body continues to burn calories after a resistance training workout as your muscles recuperate throughout the day. Furthermore, not only can anaerobic muscle-building workouts like resistance training enhance metabolism through increased EPOC, but the maintenance of lean muscle mass itself increases total daily energy expenditure by boosting BMR and, hence, overall metabolism.

Does Metabolism Decrease With Age?

Contrary to popular opinion, metabolism does not slow down as we become older. A significant study, the most comprehensive on the topic to date, was published in 2021, demonstrating that age has relatively little impact on our basal metabolic rate until the age of 60. Researchers uncovered four unique stages of metabolic life using data from approximately 6,500 persons ranging in age from 8 days to 95 years:

- From infancy through age one, when calorie burning is at its highest, the metabolic rate increases to around 50% of the adult rate.
- From the age of one to twenty, metabolism slows by roughly 3% per year.

- From the age of 20 to 60, metabolism remains constant.
- And, after the age of 60, metabolism slows by roughly 0.7% per year.

Although adults acquire a pound and a half every year on average, this weight increase cannot be linked to a slower metabolism. While metabolic rate generally declines around the age of 60, dietary and lifestyle factors are the most important contributors to weight fluctuations before this point.

What Are The Causes Of Slow Metabolism?

Looking back at the metabolic components (BMR, TEF, EAT, and NEAT), various factors can contribute to slow metabolism, some of which are controlled and others that are not.

- Height: Simply said, the smaller you are, the less energy you use, and hence the slower your BMR.
- In general, women have a slightly lower BMR than men.

- Protein has the largest thermic impact of any food (TEF), hence underrating protein will result in a slower metabolism.

- Skipping Resistance Training: Increased muscle mass equals increased metabolic rate. While all forms of movement promote general health, resistance training has a direct impact on metabolism by promoting muscle mass development and maintenance.

- Not Engaging in Intentional Exercise: If you move your body but do not engage in intentional exercise (run, workout, class, etc.), you are wasting calories.

- Limited Daily Movement: If you engage in conscious exercise but don't move your body regularly outside of the gym/run/class, you're wasting calories.

- Chronic Dieting/Calorie Deficit: Chronic undereating can result in metabolic adaptation and a drop in BMR, causing you to burn fewer calories at rest to compensate for the calorie deficit. A diet of less than 1,000 calories per day for an extended period can have a major impact on basal metabolic rate.

Fortunately, while some of the reasons are beyond your control, several are, and there are numerous strategies to enhance slow metabolism.

How Can I Fasten My Metabolism?

While many of the elements that determine metabolism are beyond our control, such as age, height, and heredity, there are numerous things we can do to enhance our metabolic rate. Although you can't "boost" your metabolism, concentrating on the aspects you can control can help you enhance your metabolic rate and overall daily energy expenditure.

1. Raise your NEAT: Consider ways to move your body more frequently outside of the gym and deliberate exercise. This will aid in increasing non-exercise activity

thermogenesis (NEAT), possibly the most underappreciated component of metabolism. Everything from playing with your children to pacing while on the phone to carrying a basket instead of a shopping cart will help you enhance your NEAT.

2. Consume More Protein: A high protein diet tends to enhance metabolism due to the high thermic effect and other variables, while it also supports the growth and maintenance of lean muscle, which helps keep BMR strong. At each meal, aim to consume at least one palm-sized serving of protein.

3. Engage in regular physical activity: Walking, cycling, dancing, skiing, or swimming regularly will help to boost your exercise activity thermogenesis (EAT), which is a factor in metabolism. Governing health agencies normally

recommend 150 minutes of moderate activity per week or 75 minutes per week.

4. Concentrate on muscle development: Prioritizing resistance and strength training can help you gain and retain more lean muscle mass, which will enhance your BMR, exercise activity thermogenesis, and total metabolism.

5. Get plenty of rest: Rest affects your energy levels, hormone balance, and hunger cues. Managing stress and prioritizing great sleep will assist in maintaining your hormones, energy levels, and metabolism robust, which is a secret weight-loss strategy.

Myths and Facts About Metabolic Energy

Let us now debunk some common metabolic fallacies and replace them with evidence-based truths:

- ❖ Myth 1: Slow metabolism cannot be changed. While genetics can influence your basic metabolism, your lifestyle choices can have a big impact on it. A balanced diet and regular physical activity, particularly strength training, can enhance your metabolism.

- ❖ Myth 2: Starvation Mode Causes Weight Loss Stalls Truth: The idea that extended calorie restriction (starvation mode) causes your metabolism to slow down greatly is rather overdone. While metabolic adaptation can occur with severe diets, this should not be used to circumvent prudent calorie decrease for weight loss.
- ❖ Myth 3: Late-night eating slows metabolism. Truth: The timing of your meals does not affect your metabolism. What is more important is the total number of calories consumed and the quality of the foods consumed.
- ❖ Myth 4: Certain foods dramatically increase your metabolism. While some

foods, such as spicy peppers or caffeine, may provide a slight and brief boost to metabolism, there are no magical foods that will drastically change your metabolism. A healthy diet and regular exercise are still your best friends.

❖ Myth 5: Metabolism Declines Rapidly with Age Truth: Metabolism declines gradually with age, not rapidly. As you become older, lifestyle choices like regular physical activity and a balanced diet become increasingly important in maintaining a healthy metabolism.

❖ Myth 6: You Can't Change Your Set Point Weight Truth: While your body has a natural range that it prefers to maintain, you can alter your set point weight with long-term lifestyle adjustments such as regular exercise and a healthy diet.

Chapter 3

Nourishing Your Body for Success

Success in a variety of spheres of life depends on taking care of your body. In addition to sustaining your physical health, proper eating is crucial for your mental and emotional well-being. Let's explore the remarkable impacts of a healthy diet on both the workplace and daily life. We'll look at how a healthy diet can boost your productivity and improve your sense of well-being. Keep Your Energy and Focus at Work You know how, after eating the right foods, you suddenly feel as if you could take on the world. Whole grains, lean proteins, and healthy fats are nutrient-dense foods that offer your body the energy it needs for a successful workday. You'll be completing jobs faster, making wiser judgments, and increasing your overall productivity at work with increased focus and mental clarity.

The Influence of Nutrient-Dense Foods

Maintaining general health and well-being requires eating a good diet. People are eating more nutrient-dense foods because they want to live healthier lives and improve their health. These foods are bursting with vitamins, minerals, and other nutrients that are vital for good health. It's a great strategy to strengthen your immune system, reduce inflammation, and promote overall well-being to include nutrient-dense foods in your diet.

Why are Foods High in Nutrients Important for a Healthy Diet?

Nutrient-dense foods are crucial in a healthy diet for a variety of reasons. Here are some major advantages of eating nutrient-rich foods daily.

- Delivers Vital Nutrients: Nutrient-dense foods give the body the nutrition it needs to function correctly. These nutrients include fiber, vitamins, minerals, and other crucial components like antioxidants. For instance, leafy green vegetables like spinach and kale are abundant in calcium, iron, and vitamins A and C. Berries and other fruits are rich sources of antioxidants, and whole grains are a source of fiber, vitamins, and minerals.

- Lowers the risk of developing chronic diseases: A diet high in nutrient-dense foods has been associated with a lower risk of developing chronic illnesses like cancer, diabetes, and heart disease. This is because certain foods contain ingredients that have anti-inflammatory characteristics and can aid the body in minimizing oxidative stress. A diet high in fruits and vegetables, for instance, has been proven to reduce the risk of heart disease and stroke.

- Supports the Management of Weight: Low in calories yet high in nutrients, nutrient-dense foods are a great option for anyone seeking to control their weight. Nutrient-dense meals allow you to eat fewer calories while still providing your body with the essential nutrients it requires. You may feel satisfied and full after eating as a result, which may help you avoid overeating.

- Improves Digestive Health: Foods that are high in nutrients are also crucial for digestive health. The high fiber content of many of these meals can aid in encouraging regular bowel movements and preventing constipation. Probiotics, a type of good bacteria that can aid in enhancing gut health, are also present in some meals that are high in nutrients.
- Increasing Energy Levels: Foods that are nutrient-rich are also crucial for sustaining energy levels throughout the day. These foods offer a consistent source of energy without elevating or lowering blood sugar

levels. For instance, nutritious grains and veggies provide complex carbs that are digested gradually and offer a consistent energy supply all day.

- Better Mental Health: Foods high in nutrients play a significant part in maintaining mental wellness. The vitamins, minerals, and other critical nutrients that support brain function, mood management, and general mental health are present in nutrient-rich diets. A balanced diet rich in nutrients can help lower the chance of mental health issues including depression, anxiety, and cognitive loss from occurring. Certain nutrients, including omega-3 fatty acids, B vitamins, magnesium, and zinc, have been demonstrated in studies to help with mood and brain function.

Nutrient-rich food Your nutritional allies.

1. Vegetables and fruits are the stars of the show. They are abundant in fiber, vitamins, minerals, and antioxidants, and help digestion as well as immunity. Your visual indication of a fruit or vegetable's nutrient density is its bright hue.

2. Whole Grains: Products like whole wheat bread, quinoa, and brown rice offer complex carbohydrates, fiber, and a range of nutrients. They gradually release energy, keeping you satisfied and energized.

3. Lean proteins are abundant in protein and necessary for muscle growth and repair. These include lean meats, poultry, fish, tofu, and lentils. They also contribute to the synthesis of hormones and enzymes.

4. Healthy Fats: Unsaturated fats are essential for heart health and brain function and may be found in foods like avocados, nuts, seeds, and olive oil. They

also facilitate the absorption of vitamins that are fat-soluble.

5. Dairy and dairy substitutes: These are sources of protein, calcium, and vitamin D. Select dairy products with reduced or no fat, or fortified non-dairy substitutes like almond or soy milk.

6. Nuts and seeds are nutritious powerhouses that include fiber, protein, healthy fats, vitamins, and minerals. A few handfuls would suffice as a snack.

7. Lean Meats To consume less saturated fat while obtaining vital amino acids use lean meat cuts.

8. Fatty Fish: Fish high in omega-3 fatty acids, such as salmon, mackerel, and sardines, provide several health advantages, including heart and brain health.

Macros: Carbs, Proteins, and Fats in Balance

To maintain total health and fitness, one must follow a balanced diet. To meet your nutrient demands and achieve your health goals, it's crucial to eat a variety of meals from all the food groups. Ensuring that you are getting the proper ratio of macro and micronutrients is also crucial. You may maximize the benefits of your diet by appropriately balancing your macro- and micronutrient intake. The significance of macronutrients and micronutrients will be covered in this blog post, along with advice on how to make sure you're receiving enough of each.

To adequately maintain the health and functioning of your body, it's crucial to make sure you consume enough of each of these macronutrients in your diet. Nutrient deficiencies can arise from eating too little of any macronutrient, whereas weight gain and other health issues can arise from eating too much of any macronutrient. Therefore, finding the ideal balance between these nutrients is crucial.

Depending on your particular demands, you may need different amounts of each macro. Your daily intake of macronutrients should consist of between 50–60% carbohydrates, 20–25% protein, and 20–30% fat. Getting the proper kinds of carbohydrates, proteins, and fats is also crucial. Lean meats, fish, nuts, and legumes are good sources of protein, while whole grains, fruits, and vegetables are good sources of carbs. Olive oil, almonds, and avocados are all good sources of fat.

You can support your body's general health and welfare by making sure you consume the proper amount and kind of each macronutrient in your diet. A well-rounded diet is built on balancing your macronutrients—carbohydrates, proteins, and fats. Each macronutrient has a specific job in supplying your body with energy and supporting its processes.

Carbohydrates are your body's primary source of energy. They offer rapid energy for workouts and daily tasks. To avoid energy crashes, the secret is to choose complex carbohydrates like whole grains, legumes, and veggies. The building blocks of life are proteins. They are necessary for some biological processes, including muscle growth and repair. Lean proteins from foods like poultry, fish, tofu, and lentils should be a part of your diet. Healthy fats are essential for overall well-being. They aid in the creation of hormones, the absorption of fat-soluble vitamins, and brain function. Among the best sources of healthy fats include avocado, almonds, seeds, and olive oil.

It is crucial to balance these macronutrients, but different people will respond best to different ratios based on their age, amount of exercise, and health objectives. Your ideal macronutrient balance can be evaluated with the aid of a certified dietitian.

Why is it crucial to keep them in balance?
The important nutrients included in a person's diet that give their body energy are referred to as macronutrients, or simply "macros." These include lipids, proteins, and carbs. Although each macronutrient plays a unique part in maintaining our health, they all work together to keep us energized and operating at our peak potential. As a result, maintaining a balance between these nutrients is crucial for our continued health.

These macronutrients give the body the energy it needs to function correctly when they are balanced. Proteins aid in the development and repair of biological tissue, carbohydrates fuel physical and mental activity, and fats fuel several bodily functions. Overall health and well-being must balance these macronutrients since doing so helps to ensure that the body can function at its peak.

In addition, regulating your macronutrient intake can aid in enhancing metabolic health. Consuming the right proportion of macronutrients helps lower cholesterol levels and lower risk factors for diabetes, heart disease, and other metabolic diseases. By upholding good eating practices, a balanced diet can assist healthy weight management.

A balanced diet also makes sure that you are obtaining adequate micronutrients or the vitamins and minerals required for healthy growth and health. Micronutrients can be found in fruits, vegetables, dairy products, and some foods that have been fortified. They serve as the fundamental building blocks for good biological functions. The body may become lacking in vital vitamins and minerals if proper levels of micronutrients aren't consumed, which could weaken the immune system and cause other health issues.

Important Micronutrients and Their Functions:

Your diet's unsung heroes are micronutrients. These are the vitamins and minerals that, despite being required by your body in smaller amounts, are just as important for overall health and well-being.

- Vitamin A is essential for maintaining healthy skin, supporting the immune system, and preserving good vision. It can be sourced from foods like spinach, carrots, and sweet potatoes.
- Vitamin C, an antioxidant, fortifies the immune system and aids in collagen production. You can find it in bell peppers, strawberries, and citrus fruits.
- Vitamin D: Essential for immune system health, mood modulation, and bone health.

found in dairy products with added vitamins and sunshine.

- Calcium is essential for healthy neuron and muscle function, strong bones, and teeth. found in leafy greens, dairy products, and non-dairy equivalents that have been fortified.
- Iron: Important for the blood's ability to carry oxygen. found in beans, fortified grains, and lean meats.
- Potassium: Helps maintain blood pressure and supports the health of the heart and muscles. found in potatoes, beans, and bananas.
- Magnesium plays a vital role in bone health, muscle and nerve function, and energy production. It is abundant in leafy greens, nuts, and seeds.
- Zinc: Crucial for DNA synthesis, wound healing, and immunological function. found in whole grains, nuts, and meat.

- Folate (Vitamin B9): Vital for the production of red blood cells and DNA. found in legumes, fortified grains, and leafy greens.
- For strong bones and proper blood clotting, vitamin K is indispensable, and it can be obtained from broccoli and leafy greens.
- Vitamin B: a class of vitamins (B1, B2, B3, B5, B6, B7, B9, and B12) involved in metabolism, generating energy, and other biological processes. a substance that is present in a variety of meals, such as whole grains, lean meats, and legumes.
- Iodine: essential for the thyroid, metabolism, and general growth. found in seafood and iodized salt.

Making sure you get enough of these vitamins and minerals is crucial. The most dependable way to meet your micronutrient demands is through a well-balanced diet full of a variety of nutrient-dense foods. Supplements may be required in some circumstances, but they should only be used with a doctor's advice.

How to Ensure You Are Getting Enough of Macro and Micronutrients

The secret is to adopt a conscious attitude when it comes to balancing your macro- and micronutrient intake. It's critical to comprehend what each vitamin works for your body before you even consider portion amounts and dietary selections. While micronutrients are necessary vitamins and minerals, macronutrients are the sources of energy.

The first step to correctly balancing these nutrients is understanding their functions in your body. When making meal and snack plans, make an effort to include complex carbohydrates, lean protein, and healthy fats in each meal and snack. Your body will have enough nutrition and energy as a result to perform at its peak throughout the day.

It's also crucial to concentrate on consuming foods high in micronutrients, such as fruits and vegetables. The vitamins and minerals found in these foods are vital for optimum health. Choose different colored fruits and vegetables to include in your diet; the more colorful, the better! Dark leafy greens, for instance, contain calcium and iron, while oranges and other citrus fruits are excellent sources of vitamin C.

You can make sure you're receiving the proper ratio of both by learning the fundamentals of macronutrients and micronutrients and including a wide variety of healthy foods in your diet. You'll have more energy and attention throughout the day as a result, in addition to preserving the health of your body.

Chapter 4

Eat Smart, Not Less

Eat Smart, Not Less is a concept that emphasizes making healthy dietary choices rather than simply consuming less food. This method emphasizes fueling your body with nutrient-dense foods rather than starvation or excessive calorie restriction. This approach is consistent with the idea that choosing healthy meals, managing portion sizes, and eating a balanced diet will lead to long-term weight loss and improved general health. It encourages people to pick whole grains, lean meats, fruits and vegetables, and healthy fats over processed foods, sweets, and empty calories. In essence, Eat Smart, Not Less is a reminder that when it comes to food, quality matters just as much as quantity, pushing for a comprehensive approach to health and weight control. It is about making informed decisions that will benefit your long-term well-being.

Portion Control and Mindful Eating

A pattern of daily food and beverage choices is the foundation of healthy eating habits. Establishing healthy eating habits benefits long-term health by increasing the intake of key nutrients that promote optimum growth and development and lowering the risk of chronic disease. High-quality, nutrient-dense foods from the five food groups—dairy, vegetables, fruits, grains, and protein—should serve as the foundation for good eating habits, and the diversity of wholesome meals available accommodates personal preferences, budgets, and cultures. While eating habits vary from person to person, basic approaches for following a balanced diet can be used. Mindfulness, or paying attention to the present moment, is a useful method for raising awareness and encouraging good eating.

With the availability of lip-smackingly delicious ready-to-eat foods on the market, our eating habits have altered considerably in recent years. In addition, because of our increasingly hectic lifestyles, we have begun to stuff ourselves with highly processed foods such as pizza, chips, cookies, desserts, aerated drinks, and items from a roadside vendor/street cafe for convenience.

This occurs occasionally owing to a lack of time, but more frequently due to easy access to certain foods and snacks. It is difficult to avoid such foods in our daily lives, but it is possible to understand how we may restrict our consumption of such processed foods by practicing portion management in our daily meals. There has been a lot of research done on the effects of big portion sizes on health.

Even when we consume healthy foods, we often feel sluggish and tired afterward, which eventually leads to extreme weight gain and poor health. When it comes to maintaining good health, losing weight, or even fighting lifestyle diseases like diabetes, hypertension, high cholesterol, and others, eating the proper portion sizes and including the right food types in our diet plays an important role.

Aside from the micro and macronutrients we consume, portion control and mindful eating are essential components of healthy nutrition. It has nothing to do with losing weight or monitoring calories. It is a healthy habit we may create to foster a pleasant relationship with our food and our bodies.

Guidelines for mindful eating
We frequently consider what foods to eat and what foods to avoid while discussing healthy eating. Have you ever considered that what you eat might not even be the most significant factor? Eat in the present moment. It entails

understanding why, when, what, where, and how much you eat.

Being in the moment and paying attention to the eating process is what is meant by mindful eating. Making healthier food choices, eating more slowly, being conscious of portion sizes, eating less by paying attention to our bodies' signals of hunger and satiety, savoring our meals more, and feeling fuller afterward are all advantages of mindful eating. Additionally, these advantages will enhance glycemic management.

Too frequently, we engage in thoughtless eating. Eating while watching TV, reading a magazine, or checking emails from work is referred to as mindless eating. Answer the following questions to determine if you are a conscious or mindless eater:

- Do you consume food rapidly (under 20 minutes)?

- Do you watch TV, talk on the phone, or use a computer while eating?
- Do you eat what's around you without thinking?
- Do you eat what is easy or readily accessible rather than making a meal plan?

You are thoughtless eating if you selected yes to any of these questions. Effective responses to these inquiries can aid you on your journey.

Hunger and Satiety: Finding the Right Balance

Understanding the delicate interaction between satisfaction and appetite is similar to learning the art of a well-performed symphony in the complex world of diet and weight management. To develop a positive relationship with food, these two seemingly opposing sensations must work together. The complicated interactions between fullness and hunger are examined in this chapter, along with the physiological and psychological variables that affect them, to help you find the perfect balance.

Satiety: The Experience of Being Full

Your body uses satiety, often known as the feeling of fullness, as a cue that enough food has been consumed. It is a complex sensation that is influenced by several physical and psychological elements.

The Satisfaction-Influencing Factors:

- Foods that are high in fiber, protein, and good fats tend to make people feel fuller longer. These nutrients promote blood sugar balance and slow digestion, which prolongs the experience of being full.
- Volume: Your level of satiety is influenced by the actual amount of food in your stomach. Fruits and vegetables, which have a high water content, might make you feel full by filling your stomach.

- Leptin, ghrelin, and insulin are important hormones in the regulation of satiety. Your brain receives a signal from leptin, often known as the "satiety hormone," telling it that you have consumed enough food. On the other side, ghrelin is referred to as the "hunger hormone" and increases appetite.

- Meal composition: The proportions of different macronutrients in a meal might affect how full you feel. Long-lasting satiety is more likely to be supported by a balanced meal that contains carbohydrates, protein, and good fats.

- Stress and Emotions: Emotional concerns can have an impact on how full you feel. Even if you are physically content, stress and emotional eating can lead to overeating.

- Put protein first: Include lean sources of protein in your diet, such as poultry, fish, tofu, and lentils. Protein aids muscle maintenance and repair in addition to increasing satiety.

- Consistently drinking water will help you stay hydrated. Sometimes, hunger and thirst are confused.

- Eat mindfully by paying attention to your food and enjoying each bite. You may recognize when you're full and avoid overeating by taking your time and eating slowly and thoughtfully.

The Body's Need for Fuel: Hunger

Your body uses hunger as a signal that it needs food. It is a fundamental and primitive sense that serves as a reminder that your body needs energy to operate at its best. However, several other elements, some of which are not completely physiological, can have an impact on appetite.

The Elements Affecting Hunger

- Blood Sugar Levels: Changes in blood sugar levels can make you feel hungry. Sugary foods and refined carbs can cause blood sugar levels to rise and fall quickly, causing hunger to return soon after eating.
- Meal Timing: Consistent meal timing can assist in controlling hunger signals. Going without food for long periods or skipping meals can make you feel more hungry.
- Psychological factors: Even when your body's energy requirements are satisfied, emotional eating, stress, and boredom can cause you to feel hungry.
- Environmental Cues: The sight, smell, and social context of food can all arouse hunger. This explains why you could get a snack appetite while dining out or viewing a food commercial.

Strategies to Manage Hunger:

- Eat frequently: Create a schedule for your meals and snacks to keep your blood sugar levels consistent and lessen your chance of experiencing extreme hunger.

- Decide on Whole Foods: Choose nutrient-dense, complete foods that help you feel full and encourage prolonged energy. Limit your intake of highly processed foods high in sugar.

- Hydrate: Sometimes, the body's hunger signs are misinterpreted as thirst signals. Stay hydrated throughout the day.

- Eat with awareness and only when you are truly hungry by paying attention to your body's hunger cues. Refrain from eating in response to external circumstances or emotional cues.

- Reduce emotional eating and decrease hunger caused by stress by implementing stress-reduction tactics such as meditation, yoga, or deep breathing exercises.

Finding the Balance: A Comprehensive Approach

It's important to nourish both your body and mind to maintain the delicate balance between satisfaction and hunger. It takes a holistic strategy that takes into account the nutritional value of your meals, your emotional eating habits, and your capacity to pay attention to your body's messages to achieve this balance.

You can develop a better relationship with food when you learn how to balance satiety and hunger. You no longer think of meals as contests to be won or lost, but rather as chances to best nourish and fuel your body. This equilibrium enables you to make food decisions that support your dietary journey and are consistent with your goals for health and well-being. The next chapter will go into more detail on how to improve your understanding of satiety and hunger and use this understanding to change the way you normally eat.

Techniques for Long-Term Weight Loss

You are not alone if you have ever started a diet to lose weight only to quickly regain it all after stopping. How do you prevent gaining weight again after all your effort? Change your focus to sustainable, long-lasting practices that will help you gradually lose weight and keep it off rather than relying on a fad diet that will only provide you with short-term results.

Hundreds of fad diets, weight-reduction regimens, and blatant scams promise quick and uncomplicated weight loss. However, a balanced, calorie-restricted diet along with increased physical activity continues to be the cornerstone of a successful weight loss program. For successful, long-term weight loss, you must alter your food and lifestyle patterns permanently. No matter why you want to lose weight, this is a fantastic moment to get started.

1. Begin by asking "Why am I overweight?"
Contrary to what you may have read, obesity is not solely a "lack of willpower" or a problem with a certain meal. In actuality, a variety of things affect what we eat. The recent changes to our surroundings and way of life make it harder to make healthy decisions, and we prefer to eat more prepared or takeout meals. Compared to home-cooked meals, this typically means more fat, sugar, and salt, as well as frequently greater serving sizes.

At the same time, we are exercising less than earlier generations. We spend less time walking or riding bicycles and spend more time sitting down while working and enjoying ourselves. We've lost the chance to exercise on the way to work because many of us are working from home more frequently these days.
You can lower your chance of having heart and circulation disease by up to 35% by increasing your level of physical activity.

Consider the possible causes of your weight gain as a good starting point. Is this a fresh development or a recurring pattern? Did you start acting differently around the time you started gaining weight, such as dining out more, being less active, or consuming different foods? If you're unsure of where you're making mistakes, try maintaining a food and drink journal for a week in a notebook or tracking your meals on a smartphone app.

2. Set a goal for losing weight.

It might be tough to lose weight. Determine how much weight you want to lose first. How we define a "healthy weight" may skew when more people become overweight. Your body mass index (BMI) is a calculation of how much you weigh with how tall you are. If you are aware of these figures, you can calculate your BMI and target weight using a free online calculator.

Don't be discouraged or feel you have to take drastic actions if you weigh more than you thought. Divide it up into manageable steps, and concentrate on each one. Aim to lose 10% of your body weight if you need to lose a lot of weight. Even if you remain overweight later, this will have significant positive effects on your health and may seem more attainable. If it will take some time for you to reach your ideal weight, don't give up. It probably took a very long time to gradually start.

3. Make adjustments that fit your lifestyle.

There are a plethora of diets, products, and meals that promise to make us lose weight. Despite these confusing options, the fundamental rule of weight loss is straightforward: You must consume fewer calories than you expend. Beyond that, each person will respond differently to different diets, with choosing a plan you can follow is one of the most important considerations. Discovering the path that is best for you is crucial.

Many people find it beneficial to avoid thinking about "diets" in favor of a long-term, lifestyle-compatible strategy. Some people find that cutting back on fat or carbohydrates is effective, while others choose to watch calories or reduce their calorie consumption on particular days. You risk depriving yourself of necessary nutrients if your regimen is too tight and eliminates entire food groups.

4. Consume a healthy diet.

Your favorite foods may be available in reduced-calorie, low-calorie, or light variations. However, don't assume that this means they are also low in salt and sugar. Check food labels and attempt to choose healthy options rather than just those with fewer calories. Maintaining even a slight weight decrease over the long run is healthy for your health and something to be proud of. You don't have to eliminate all high-calorie meals because some of them provide beneficial elements, such as oily salmon, unsalted almonds, and avocado. However, you might wish to consume them less frequently or in smaller quantities.

5. Keep going even if improvement is slow.

It may take some time to reach your "ideal" weight, and there may be times when it seems impossible. If your weight reduction is slow or you reach a plateau, don't get discouraged. Maintaining even a slight weight decrease is admirable and good for your health in the long run. Keep going, then!

Chapter 5

Superfoods for Super Metabolism

Metabolism-boosting meals may aid in weight loss. However, foods that can speed up your metabolism and burn fat do not ensure that you will lose weight. You must still do your share. If you're attempting to lose or keep weight off, you might be seeking foods that improve your metabolism.

Your metabolic rate can be slightly increased by eating certain meals. This is the amount of calories your body has expended. Including these foods in your diet may aid in your goal of reducing body fat or preventing excessive weight gain. However, increasing your intake of certain foods won't always result in weight loss. To help with weight loss, they should be used as a supplement to a well-balanced, moderately calorie-restricted diet.

Metabolism-Boosting Foods Revealed

1. Quinoa: Quinoa may look similar to cous cous, but it is far superior. It has about three times the amount of (complete) protein and is also a complex carbohydrate. This makes it ideal for bulking up salads for lunch and staving off tummy rumbles late into the afternoon. To save time and money, buy it already cooked.

2. Avocado: For far too long, fat has been demonized. We need fat not only to burn fat but also to keep our brains happy and to be the king of satiety. One study published in Nutrition Journal found that eating half an avocado with lunch reduced hunger by 40% for the next two hours. Avocado isn't just for lunch; try it with breakfast to satisfy your mid-morning biscuit cravings!

3. Lentils: It takes longer to chew a tablespoon of lentils, so imagine how long it takes to digest them! This is because of their high fiber content, which means they will keep you fuller for longer. Lentils are a high-density, low-calorie food, making them ideal for weight loss. Not to mention they're high in energy-producing iron, which is needed for those extra gym sessions!

4. Rice (brown): Simply change fluffy, white rice for its nuttier counterpart to lower the GI of your meal and stabilize your blood sugar level. Brown rice is what white rice used to look like before the fibrous hull was removed. In terms of nutritional content, it's far fleshier than white rice, as it's high in B vitamins and minerals like calcium, magnesium, and potassium.

5. Water: You've probably heard that drinking water with your meal would make you feel fuller faster. However, a

study from Pennsylvania State University discovered that having the same quantity of water in a soup with your meal rather than as a drink causes you to eat less of that meal and less throughout the day! What better way to put your leftover vegetables to use?

6. Eggs: Forget everything you thought you knew about eggs. They are not the cause of elevated cholesterol, but they are nutritious powerhouses and one of the greatest protein sources available, ranking high on the Satiety Index scale. Hard-boiled eggs are the ideal pre-packaged snack; just leave the shell on until the very last minute to prevent irritating sensitive office nostrils!

7. Green Leafy Vegetables: Kale, spinach, Swiss chard, and other dark green leafy vegetables are low in calories yet high in fiber. Using leafy greens, you can double (or triple) the size of your meal without

double the calories. You will, however, increase your intake of body-friendly nutrients and antioxidants! Pack them into salads, melt them into pasta, or shred them into stir-fries and curries.

8. Yogurt from Greece: Put down the fruit-flavored 'diet' yogurt and head to the Greek! It may add a few extra calories at first, but it has significantly more protein and far less sugar. You should try to consume more protein to help with appetite control, muscle mass preservation, and general calorie-zapping powers. As a post-workout snack, try a few heaping teaspoons sprinkled with fresh fruit to calm your muscles and keep that 'after cardio' appetite at bay.

9. Chipotle peppers: Hot spices and herbs are thermogenic. This means they stimulate thermogenesis, which is a mechanism within the body that converts calories to heat, allowing us to use them more

quickly. Enough said; start seasoning your meals!

10. Porridge: When it comes to weight loss, cutting out carbs is a frequent diet fallacy. Carbohydrates are necessary for optimum brain function and give energy, which is necessary if you want to make that HIIT session count! Stick to complex carbohydrates like oatmeal for longer-lasting energy. A bowl of oats before bed will help you balance your blood sugar levels and sleep peacefully till morning. Their high phosphorus level (which can be amplified by adding a spoonful of mixed seeds) also aids in muscle rehabilitation.

11. Cinnamon: This warming, sweet super spice regulates blood sugar levels, which can help to reduce a sweet tooth. In place of honey, generously shake over oats or yogurt!

12. Chickpeas: Researchers in Australia invited a group of volunteers to include chickpeas in their daily diet for 12 weeks. The subjects ate less food, particularly grains, throughout the three months they were fed chickpeas! Add these knobbly legumes to your stews and soups like our Australian friends. Blend with some decent olive oil, lemon juice, and garlic to make quick homemade hummus.

13. Dark Chocolate: Does consuming chocolate result in weight loss? Not exactly. However, denying yourself what you enjoy will not work in the long run. The key to this one is damage limitation - In the evening, a few pieces of high-quality dark chocolate will not only satisfy your sweet craving but will also provide you with heart-healthy flavonoids and cholesterol-lowering nutrients!

14. Popcorn: By substituting this movie favorite for crisps, you will not only

consume fewer calories, but you will also improve heart health and protect against age-related disease, thanks to the polyphenols and antioxidant characteristics of the magnificent popped corn!

15. The seeds of chia: These stylish little seeds sprout miraculously in water (and in your stomach!), keeping you full for hours. It's not magic; it's a lot of indigestible fiber! Chia seeds have a high carbohydrate content, but because the bulk of those carbs are fiber, you won't experience the same insulin surge as you would with a typical high-carb diet. Put them on your muesli or in a smoothie for a filling snack.

16. Cooked potatoes (cold): When white, boiled potatoes cool, they produce a large amount of resistant starch, a material similar to fiber that keeps you satisfied for a long time. Make a frittata with your

leftover boiled tatties for a satisfying breakfast or hearty lunch.

17. Xylitol: Artificial sweeteners, in general, should be avoided at all costs. They are not only chemically loaded, but they also do little to curb sugar cravings because they continue to disrupt your blood sugar levels. However, xylitol, an extract from the South American stevia plant that is considerably more natural than its name implies, contains no calories, is 300 times sweeter than sugar, has no impact on blood sugar, and even aids in tooth whitening!

18. Fatty fish: Salmon, mackerel, trout, and herring are well-known for their anti-inflammatory good fats. They also include iodine, a nutrient necessary for a properly functioning thyroid, which is responsible for the proper operation of your metabolism.

19. Cruciferous vegetables, such as broccoli, cauliflower, and Brussels sprouts, are strong in fiber and contain more protein than water-based salad vegetables. Try roasting them and adding them to salads, or keep them raw and dip them in hummus!

Including Superfoods in Your Everyday Diet: There is no single food that provides all of the nutrition, energy, and health advantages that your body requires to stay healthy. Your body needs a variety of vitamins, minerals, and nutrients to function properly, which is why it's critical to watch what you eat. Incorporating antioxidant-rich superfoods (chemicals that combat genetic alterations and cancer-causing tissue damage) can help to reduce cell damage. If you incorporate some of these superfoods into your regular diet, you can be confident that your body is receiving the nutrients it requires to thrive.

1. Make a Spirulina Smoothie: According to
   a study conducted by the University of
   Maryland Medical Center, spirulina, a
   blue-green algae, is rich in nutrients that
   can help avoid harm and stress to your
   body. The powdery ingredient improves
   your immune system, but it's not the
   easiest thing to incorporate into your
   morning routine. Solve the problem by
   requesting your favorite smoothie shop to
   include it in your green smoothie.

2. Steel-cut Oatmeal with Walnuts: This
   superfood double whammy is incredibly
   simple to make, especially during the
   colder months when all you want is
   something warm. Walnuts are the
   heart-healthiest of all tree nuts, according
   to University Hospitals of Cleveland.
   They include vital omega-3 fatty acids
   that help your heart function properly.
   Add a handful to a bowl of steel-cut oats
   to help decrease cholesterol while also

providing protein to keep you satiated for longer.

3. Vinaigrette with Apple Cider Vinegar: What is ACV incapable of? But if you're stuck wondering how to utilize it, a simple change is to replace it with the white vinegar you use in vinaigrettes. Apple cider vinegar aids digestion, alkalizes the body to aid in nutrient absorption, and has anti-inflammatory qualities.

4. A handful of nuts can be added to your pesto: Nut consumption has been related to living longer and healthier lives, according to a big study published in the New England Journal of Medicine. While traditional pestos are created with pine nuts, you can always add a handful of your favorite tree nuts to boost the antioxidant content of your sauce. To increase the flavor, toast them before tossing them in.

5. Replace the sugar with canned pumpkin: This is a fat swap, not a sugar exchange; canned pumpkin may replace the eggs and oil (called fats) in your baked goods while still keeping them fluffy and light. If you're having a cheat day and want to create brownies, cookies, cakes, or other treats, consider this substitution to boost your Beta-carotene and anti-inflammatory compounds while minimizing your calorie intake.

6. Dress your salads with pure maple syrup: If you must use a sweetener in your salad dressings, choose something natural, such as pure maple syrup. According to a study published in the Journal of Agriculture and Food Chemistry, it is high in polyphenols, which have been demonstrated to improve brain function and health. However, keep in mind that a sweetener is still a sweetener, so use it carefully.

7. In place of sour cream, use Greek yogurt in your soups: In the winter, nothing beats a hearty cup of soup or chili to warm the soul. However, foods high in cream and dairy products can be bad for both your stomach and your waistline. University Hospitals recommends substituting Greek yogurt for heavy creams since it has more protein, probiotics, and vitamin D than plain yogurt.

8. Popcorn with Nutritional Yeast: The B-complex vitamins in nutritional yeast (called "nooch") are an easy method to add zinc, folates, niacin, and other minerals to your diet. For a flavor boost, sprinkle it over popcorn instead of butter and cheese; it will remind you of Parmesan cheese. You'll also get a substantial (vegetarian!) serving of protein, fiber, and B-12.

9. Toss a Handful of Blueberries Into Your Breakfast: Dark berries, such as

blueberries, are not only lower in sugar than other fruits, but they are also high in anthocyanins, which are anti-bacterial and anti-inflammatory. The Society for the Study of Ingestive Behavior discovered that eating blueberries helped keep blood glucose constant in a study. Blueberries are one of our favorites because they're so simple to add to overnight oats for a little sweetness and a lot of nutrition.

10. Cauliflower puree can be used to thicken soups: All cruciferous vegetables contain cancer-fighting chemicals, but cauliflower is especially high in vitamins C, K, and folate. Making pizza crusts, breads, and other carbs from cauliflower has grown trendy, but it is time-consuming. Instead, use pureed cauliflower as a thickening in soups for an easy, no-mess approach to increase your nutrient intake.

11. In Brownies, replace the sugar with unsweetened applesauce: Unsweetened

applesauce is not only a terrific sugar substitute, but it also has far fewer calories. Apples are high in vitamin C, potassium, and fiber, all of which help get things moving in your digestive tract. Include the apple skin, which is said to have at least double the antioxidant potential of the apple meat.

12. Salad with flakes of canned salmon: The omega-3 fatty acids in salmon are extremely beneficial to heart health, but we understand that cooking a piece of salmon for your daily salad can be quite a task. Instead of dry grilled chicken, seek for canned, line-caught, high-quality salmon to rapidly flake into salads. You'll have a filling, delicious lunch that isn't as routine.

13. Carrots can be hidden in baked goods: Carrots include antioxidants known as carotenoids, which have been linked to improved eye health and a lower risk of

prostate cancer. They can be stealthily grated into baked items for a covert boost or even added to sauces for a hint of sweetness.

14. Salads can benefit from the addition of roasted tomatoes: Tomatoes are notorious for their acidity, yet they are high in lycopene, which has been found in some studies to protect against breast and prostate cancer. They also contain a lot of beta-carotene. Roast them in olive oil to bring out the flavor, and your workday salad will become suddenly more gourmet.

15. Serve your salad with shelled edamame: Edamame is a popular pre-meal snack in Japanese restaurants, but it's also a great vegetarian source of protein, as well as vitamins A and C. Add shelled edamame to your salad for a unique twist.

16. Make Salsa with Black Beans: Black beans, like all beans, are an excellent

source of lysine and other vital amino acids. Because they are plant-based proteins, your kidneys, and cardiovascular system will appreciate how easy they are to utilize in the body, especially when compared to animal-based proteins. Black beans not only have a high protein content, but they also have a high concentration of disease-fighting phytochemicals and fiber—the two most important food groups to focus on in a healthy diet.

17. Sunflower seeds can be used in place of croutons: If you're craving crunch in your salad, try a handful of sunflower seeds instead of croutons. Sunflower seeds include magnesium, which can help with digestion as well as irritation and stress.

18. Flaxseeds Can Be Added to Pancake Batter: Flaxseeds are an excellent egg substitute since they are high in omega-3 fatty acids and fiber." To add nutrients to

your pancake batter, simply combine ground flax seeds with water. You won't notice the difference in your weekend pancake indulgence - you can also sprinkle them on top of your stack of pancakes for a slightly crispy accent.

19. Place the Kiwi in the Sparkling Water: Kiwis are a low-calorie alternative to pre-bottled effervescent drinks, which may include significant amounts of sugar. To make your own, slice kiwi and dip it into sparkling water. A kiwi has more potassium than a banana and is high in both soluble and insoluble fiber.

20. Instead of coffee, drink tea: For some, this may be the simplest trade of all; for coffee addicts, perhaps not so much. However, the advantages of drinking calorie-free, low-cost, and delicious tea are considerable. It can help with blood pressure, osteoporosis, heart health, and so much more.

Metabolic Health Recipes and Meal Plans

Whether you begin a 7-day or 10-day diet plan, you will still require a precise meal plan. It must include meals from all food categories to achieve your nutritional requirements. Because of this, you should seek professional assistance while developing such tight diet plans. Here are some free meal plan ideas to get you started on your metabolic diet plan:

Day 1

Breakfast

- 1 cup of standard coffee
- 1/2 cup shredded wheat with 1 cup 1% milk
- 1 medium slice whole-wheat bread, 2 teaspoons regular jelly
- 1/3 cup orange juice

Lunch

- 1 apple, medium
- Two medium slices of whole-wheat bread, two ounces of unseasoned roast beef,

three slices of tomato, one lettuce leaf, and one teaspoon of low-calorie mayonnaise make a roast beef sandwich.

- A single cup of water

Dinner

- 2 ounces of salmon cooked in 1 1/2 teaspoons of vegetable oil
- A half cup of green beans
- 1 white dinner roll, tiny
- One teaspoon of margarine on three-quarters of a medium-baked potato
- 1 cup unsweetened iced tea
- 2 cups of water

Snack

- Two and a half cups of popcorn seasoned with a quarter teaspoon of margarine

Day 2:

Breakfast: Scrambled egg with spinach and tomato

Lunch: Tuna salad with lettuce, tomato, and cucumber for lunch

Dinner: Roasted Mediterranean veggies, puy lentils, and tahini dressing for dinner

Snack: boiled egg on pita bread

Day 3

Breakfast muffin stuffed with eggs and vegetables

Lunch consists of vegetable soup and two oatcakes.

Baked sweet potato, chicken breast, and lush green vegetables for dinner

Carrot sticks and hummus as a snack

Day 4

Breakfast: Oatmeal with honey, raisins, and frozen blueberries served with a cup of orange juice

Lunch: tuna and cucumber wrap, boiled egg, and 1/4 cup of low-fat vanilla yogurt

Dinner: Spaghetti with homemade tomato sauce, dark green veggies, and lean meatballs (a vegetarian equivalent is available).

Snacks include whole-grain crackers or carrot sticks with hummus.

Day 5

Breakfast: mashed avocado and cooked egg on rye toast

Broccoli quinoa with toasted almonds for lunch

Sesame salmon, purple sprouting broccoli, and sweet potato mash for dinner

Tangerine with Brazil nuts as a snack

Chapter 6

Overcoming Plateaus and Challenges

Losing weight requires a significant level of motivation, at least at first. You kickstart yourself into high gear right away, by going to the gym regularly and eating nutritious foods. If you master the balance of calories in and calories out, you'll start to lose weight quickly. Every time you step off the scale in the morning, you could do a mini victory dance. These small glimpses of achievement may be enough to motivate you even more than you were before.

But, inevitably, success begins to slow. You're still doing everything correctly—the gym has become your second home, and you've consumed an inordinate amount of nuts. But, day after day, weigh-in after weigh-in, the same number appears on that stupid little screen. You haven't altered anything about your behavior, so why isn't the weight coming off? Is the scale malfunctioning?

The plateau not only hinders your weight reduction progress, but it can also kill your motivation. Seeing the same number over and over is reason enough to decelerate your once-inspiring roll. You might be more willing to skip the gym on days when you don't feel like going, or you might be more tempted to take advantage of that free cookie at the company birthday celebration. While it is disappointing when your fat loss slows, reaching a weight loss plateau is entirely natural and even expected.

What exactly is a weight-loss plateau?
A weight-loss plateau occurs when your weight does not change. Everyone who attempts to lose weight ultimately finds themselves at a weight-loss plateau. Even still, most people are astonished when this happens to them because

they continue to eat healthily and exercise consistently. Even well-planned weight-loss efforts can halt, which is a frustrating truth.

What factors contribute to a weight-loss plateau?

A quick dip is usual during the first few weeks of reducing weight. This is due, in part, to the fact that when you first restrict calories, the body obtains essential energy by releasing glycogen stores. Glycogen is a carbohydrate that is found in the muscles and the liver. Glycogen is partially composed of water. When glycogen is burnt for energy, it releases water, resulting in largely water-weight loss. However, this impact is just transient.

Both muscle and fat are lost as you lose weight. Your metabolism (the rate at which you burn calories) is maintained with help from muscle. Since your metabolism slows down when you lose weight, you end up burning less calories than you did when you were heavier. Your slowed metabolism will reduce your weight loss even if you consume the same quantity of calories that made you lose weight. When the number of calories you burn and consume equals one another, you enter a plateau.

You must either raise your physical activity level or cut calories if you want to shed more weight. Even though it won't result in greater weight reduction, sticking to your previous weight loss plan may help you keep it.

Managing Weight Loss Stalls

To break through a weight loss plateau, you must either eat less or exercise more. This may be easier said than done depending on other things such as your sleep schedule or stress levels. However, it is feasible to lose fat after reaching a weight loss plateau. Here are some suggestions to help you get back on track.

1. Keep an eye out for Post-Workout
   Overeating: You've earned the right to eat
   extra after a hard workout, right? And,
   after all, don't you need to refuel? That
   mindset, on the other hand, can stymie
   your weight loss efforts. You could run
   five miles longer, but it's really simple to
   reward yourself with more than 500
   calories. The satisfaction usually far
   outweighs the extra calories burned.

   These extra calories add up: If you
   consume a 500-calorie treat many times
   each week, you could be consuming an
   extra day's worth of calories per week or
   more than 6,000 calories per month. That
   can make a significant difference.

2. Don't overestimate your level of activity:
   When you start working out more, you
   may encounter a condition known as
   compensatory inactivity. That instance,
   you may be exercising more yet moving

less during the day. Many people develop the habit of keeping score. During your morning sweat session, you busted your butt. When you go home, you sit down on the couch for the rest of the day to binge-watch your favorite Netflix show because you've already accomplished enough for the day. That's a mistake: if you're serious about maintaining your weight loss, getting into the habit of not moving after exercising can be detrimental.

Furthermore, including more activity throughout your day will help you stay motivated. Make an effort to be active whenever possible—take your dog for a walk, play soccer with your kids, throw an impromptu dance party, or set a daily step count goal for yourself.

3. The Correct Way to Fuel Up: Maintaining a high-intensity routine increases your hunger. You can feel ravenous after your workout, causing you to overeat and instantly gain all of those calories back. So play the precautionary game: If you're hungry before your workout, chances are you'll be hungry afterward. Consider having a pre-workout snack to satisfy your hunger. You don't want something too heavy or rich, which can make you feel bloated. Instead, reach for an apple, which is high in simple carbohydrates and will provide you with energy, or a handful of almonds, which are high in beneficial fats and protein and will satisfy your appetite.

4. Maintain Consistency in the Gym: When it comes to losing that last bit of weight, consistency is everything. According to a British study, missing just one workout increases your chances of missing another

by 61 percent. This does not imply that you must be a workout perfectionist, but it does emphasize the need for hard work over time. Consistency is also important in your regimen. Regardless of what you may hear. A fat loss program can only work if you adhere to a routine long enough to learn it.

The sooner you master a workout, the better you will become at it. That means you may add more weight to it, which will help you grow and keep muscle, allowing you to burn more calories throughout the day and fight fat. Then, usually after 4 to 6 weeks, you can consider varying your exercises. Once you've mastered the fundamentals, you can on to more difficult varictics, such as alternating the classic flat bench press with the incline or close-grip bench press.

5. Reduce your stress and sleep more: When the scale refuses to budge, people should look at more than simply their diets. It might be time to turn on your sleep tracker as well. Worrying more and getting less than six hours of sleep per night can hurt your waistline. This is because stress and sleep disrupt hormone function and raise cortisol levels, both of which are linked to excess weight and belly fat.

6. Keeping a Food Journal: Many people attribute their weight loss success to maintaining food journals since it provide a clear insight into their dietary habits. People frequently believe they have reached a weight reduction plateau despite maintaining the same diet, exercise routine, and sleep patterns, but this isn't necessarily the case.

Maintaining a healthy calorie deficit, eating good meals, and getting adequate sleep and water can dramatically lower the risk of plateauing. While tracking your exercises, calories, and sleep may not be for everyone, it can help dieters retain consistency. Be cautious, though, as this habit may lead to harmful eating patterns in certain people; avoid it if you find yourself becoming unduly obsessive.

7. Appropriate Caloric Intake: You might progressively become acclimated to consuming fewer calories because your body adapts to the energy it receives. If you consume only 1,200 calories per day on a constant basis, which is not recommended for most people, your body will adjust to functioning on that lower calorie intake. This is why dietitians recommend decreasing weight gradually.

8. Hydration is essential: Water is essential for many body functions, including weight regulation. Dehydration can cause your body to confuse the need for water with hunger, increasing the urge to eat rather than reach for your water bottle. Staying hydrated allows you to feel fuller for longer. According to a 2016 study, well-hydrated people had a lower BMI than those who were not appropriately hydrated.

9. Reduce your alcohol consumption: Your favorite alcoholic beverages may have more calories than you know; for example, a margarita may contain up to 300 calories. Aside from the calorie content, alcohol might boost overall food consumption. Craft beers, which can have up to 300 calories per can, should be avoided. If you've reached a weight loss

plateau, try cutting back on alcohol or switching to lower-calorie options.

Causes of Emotional Eating

Almost everything can arouse an urge to eat. Workplace stress and financial anxiety are two prominent external reasons for emotional eating. Health issues and relationship issues can also contribute to People who follow strict diets or have a history of dieting and are more likely to eat emotionally. Other probable internal causes include a lack of introspective awareness (being aware of how you feel). Alexithymia (inability to understand, interpret, or explain emotions) Emotion dysregulation (inability to handle emotions) inverted hypothalamic pituitary adrenal (HPA) stress axis (underactive cortisol response to stress)

How to Stop Emotional Eating

It can be difficult to break a habit like emotional eating, but it is achievable. Here are some coping strategies.

❖ **Begin a diary of your emotions.**

The more you understand your habits, the better. Eating in response to emotion might be automatic. The more you understand how you feel when you do particular things, the better your chances of altering them. Keep track of the occasions when you eat yet are not physically hungry. Make a note of what was going on, how you were feeling, and any emotions you noted when you felt the impulse to eat.

You could also wish to include a space to write down what you did. Did you eat right away? Did you wait a few minutes? Did you do anything to distract yourself? Try not to judge yourself based on your results. Try to be truly curious about what happens when you eat in response to emotions. This requires a lot of practice. Be gentle with yourself as you begin your exploration. It doesn't have to be perfect.

❖ **Find alternative means of coping.**
You can start making changes once you've learned more about the emotions, situations, or thoughts that can lead to bingeing. If you observe that you always eat when you are stressed, it is the stress that has to be addressed. Consider some stress-relieving activities. If you realize that you eat when you're bored, think about strategies to deal with your boredom. What else might you do to pass the time? It takes effort and practice to change your thinking from grabbing food to engaging in other activities. Experiment with several things to determine what works best for you.

❖ **Incorporate Physical Activities**

Moving your body can be a very effective technique to deal with stress and anxiety. Physical activity helps to lower stress hormone levels in the body. Endorphins are also released, which elevate your mood. In order to address underlying emotional eating triggers, an exercise regimen can be helpful. Not everything has to be intense. Try going for a five-minute stroll or doing some mild stretching if you aren't already active. Note your reaction and how it affects you.

❖ **Try mindfulness.**

Mindfulness practices such as yoga appear to have an additional advantage. People who regularly practice yoga report lower levels of stress and anxiety. Mindfulness offers numerous advantages for mental health. It is an effective strategy for controlling anxiety and sadness. It has also been demonstrated to minimize stress eating. Mindfulness is the discipline of paying attention to the current moment. If you find that stress, depression, or worry are triggers for your eating, mindfulness activities may be beneficial.

Plan your meals

Planning your meals can help you maintain a cooler or neutral state. Meal planning is associated with increased food diversity, higher diet quality, and lower obesity. Meal planning does not require you to prepare food for a week. Instead, consider creating a weekly meal plan that includes breakfast, lunch, dinner, and a snack. Then, pick when you will eat each meal. Consider your next scheduled meal if you have a strong desire to eat. It could only be a half-hour drive. Consider how long you can go without eating. Try not to plan meals too close to bedtime, and keep all of your meals within a

12-hour window, such as 7:00 a.m. to 7:00 p.m. This means you should eat every 3 hours.

Distractions must be avoided.

When you eat while working or watching TV, your brain misses out on the complete eating experience. When you eat, pay your complete attention to the meal if feasible. This can improve your appreciation of the cuisine. When you are preoccupied, you are more inclined to consume faster. It takes time for your stomach to signal to your brain that you're full. If you eat quickly, you may be consuming more than your body requires before your brain can warn you to stop.

How to Maintain Motivation and Focus Throughout Your Journey

Losing weight can be a difficult endeavor that takes commitment, focus, and drive. Starting a weight loss journey is simple, but remaining motivated to attain your objectives is a whole different story. If you're having trouble staying motivated and focused on your path, here are some pointers to help.

1. Set attainable goals: Setting reasonable objectives and writing them down will help you attain them and contribute to improved health later in life. Goal-setting is an art, and SMART goals can help you get it correctly. SMART objectives are:

   - Instead of "lose weight," make your aim something like "lose 15 pounds by eating healthier foods and working out five times a week."

   - Measurable: How will you track your progress? Weigh-ins every day or every week? Do you keep track of your meals and activities?

   - Attainable: Set goals that are a little outside of your comfort zone but not impossible to achieve. If you know you don't have time to exercise for an hour every day, seven days a week, don't make that your objective.

- Realistic: Realistic goals are long-term objectives. Losing 30 pounds in a month is an unrealistic aim. Losing one to two pounds every week is doable.

- Timely: Set a completion deadline for your goals—divide your major goal (reduce 15 pounds) into smaller milestones with a due date: Lose five pounds per month for three months.

Be adaptable in your ambitions. If you discover that you will not be able to complete your objective by the deadline you set for yourself, it is acceptable to extend the deadline—or even revise your aims.

2. Keep track of your food intake and physical activity: Recording what you eat and how much you exercise boosts your attentiveness and helps you remain on track with your goals. It aids in determining what works best and what may not. Knowing you'll be writing

down what you eat and when you exercise motivates you to make healthier choices in the present. You will also learn a lot about the nutritional value of the foods you eat, which can help you make better judgments. You can track your diet and activity in a variety of methods, including:

- Use an old-fashioned pen and paper.
- Add the information to a text-editing or note-taking software.
- Use a goal-tracking or food-tracking app.
- Wear a personal fitness tracker and download the tracker's app to establish and monitor your goals, measure your food and drink intake, and set reminders.

3. Use positive self-talk: Nobody can inspire you as well as you can. Your thoughts matter, as does the way you communicate with yourself. Be gentle and understanding. Don't berate yourself if you miss an exercise. Instead, remark, "It's okay; things happen." Instead, I'll commit to working out

tomorrow." If you eat a doughnut, be gracious about it: "I can enjoy unhealthy food now and then because I'm playing a long game." Change thinking like "this is too difficult" into "this is so difficult, but I know I'm up for the challenge. Avoid sayings like I should work out today and I need to eat better today. Say something like, I want to exercise today (or consume healthy food today) so that I can achieve my goals.

4. Create a to-do list or a calendar: Set up a physical or virtual calendar or a daily or weekly checklist that coincides with your SMART goals if lists, checklists, and calendars inspire you. On your schedule and/or checklist, use particular language. Write "Walk for 30 minutes at 3:00 PM" instead of "Walk." Knowing how good it feels to cross something off your list may be all the drive you need on bad days.

5. Maintain a weight-loss journal: Writing in a journal allows you to stay connected to your

weight-loss thoughts and emotions. The main thing is to write in the notebook and reflect on the day to help you move cluttered thoughts, ideas, and emotions from your brain to a physical place to help you clear your mind. A notebook can help you spot trends in your life—perhaps you realize that when you don't get enough sleep, you're less inspired to exercise, or you notice that when you're stressed, you're more prone to binge eating. Keeping a journal can help you stay focused and motivated.

6. Engage in hobbies and eat foods that you enjoy: Walking, running, and lifting weights are not the only forms of physical activity. When it comes to exercise, you have a lot of alternatives, many of which don't even feel like exercise. Find activities that you enjoy, and you'll be more inspired to participate in them. Similarly, don't go on a "diet" that requires you to consume only melba bread and salad. Begin by making a list of things

you enjoy eating, and then move down the list making notes on how you may include them into your diet. For example, if you enjoy rich, creamy pasta meals, create calorie-conscious substitutes or serve your favorite pasta as a side dish to consume a smaller portion.

7. Find a fitness or weight-loss buddy: A friend or family member who is also trying to lose weight might be one of your most powerful allies—and strongest motivators. Working out with a partner makes it more enjoyable, the time flies by, and you feel less alone in your weight-loss journey. When you and your workout partner are not feeling it, you may assist in motivating each other and holding each other accountable, increasing your likelihood of sticking to your training schedule and healthy eating plan.

8. Rejoice in Small Victories Celebrate your minor victories along the way. Weight loss is a process, and it's crucial to celebrate the

minor triumphs along the road. Have you lost any weight this week? It's a reason to rejoice! Have you taken a stroll every day this week? It's a reason to rejoice! Treat Yourself to Reward yourself when you achieve your objectives. Get a massage, a new dress, or a night out with friends. Giving yourself a reward can keep you motivated and provide you with something to look forward to.

9. Never Give Up Finally, never quit. Remember that setbacks are common and that having terrible days is OK. Allow one bad day or setback to destroy your entire journey. Continue to press on while remembering why you started in the first place.

Remember that a weight reduction journey is about making lifestyle changes that will help you maintain a healthy weight in the long run, not just reducing weight. This includes implementing good habits into your everyday routine, such as eating a balanced diet, exercising regularly, and managing stress. Don't just think about the number on the scale; think about how you feel as well. Do you have more stamina? Do you sleep better now? Are you able to participate in things that you couldn't before? Non-scale successes are just as essential as scale victories and can help keep you motivated and on track.

To summarize, staying motivated during a weight loss journey necessitates effort, commitment, and tenacity. Set reasonable objectives, discover your why, appreciate tiny victories, keep a journal, surround yourself with people who support you, reward yourself, and never give up. Remember that every journey begins with a single step, so take that first step and keep going.

Conclusion

We've come to the conclusion of our trip together in "Chow Down, Slim Up: Beat Your Diet with Eating Right," and I hope you can now see that the road to long-term health and sustainable weight management is not built with shame, deprivation, or restrictive diets. It's an adventure in self-empowerment, exploration, and self-compassion.

You have studied the science of metabolism in great detail, learned the benefits of mindful eating, and discovered the fascinating world of nutrient-dense foods. You've come to appreciate the harmony of macronutrients and the critical function of micronutrients in your health.

But keep in mind that this is a new beginning, not just a conclusion. With knowledge in hand, you're prepared to make decisions that fit your own goals and physique. You now have the means to change your relationship with food such that it is one of nourishing, contentment, and vitality.

Never has "Chow Down, Slim Up" been about taking cheap corners or quick cures. The goal has been to illuminate the way to a lifetime of wellness. The goal is the lively, healthy life you've imagined for yourself, not a particular dress size or weight.

So, proceed with assurance. Savor every delicious, nutrient-rich bite and treasure the renewed vitality that fills your days as you embrace the delight of eating healthfully. You have the ability to make decisions that will not only enable you to lose those excess pounds but also enable you to flourish in every area of your life.

This is the first step on your path to a healthier, more attractive, and more fit self. Thank you for taking part in "Chow Down, Slim Up."